POWERFUL NATURAL REMEDIES FOR JOINT PAIN

Natural Solutions to Relieve and Treat Joint Pain

Taylor Francis

DISCLAIMER

TABLE OF CONTENT

Enhance Your Knowledge: Exploring Additional Resources and References

Chapter 7

CONCLUSION

INTRODUCTION

Synopsis of Joint Pain

A prevalent ailment that impacts millions of people globally is joint discomfort. It describes pain, soreness, or inflammation in the body's joints, including the wrists, shoulders, hips, and knees. Numerous factors, such as arthritis, trauma, overuse, or certain medical disorders, may cause joint discomfort.

This section offers a thorough explanation of joint pain, including its origins, signs, and implications for day-to-day functioning. Through exploring the many varieties of joint pain and their unique attributes, readers will get an all-encompassing understanding of this common ailment.

The Value of Natural Treatments

Natural therapies are becoming more and more popular for treating joint pain because of their low side effects and possible advantages. To relieve joint pain and enhance general joint health, natural treatments include using materials that may be found in nature, such as herbs, essential oils, nutritional supplements, and physical therapy.

The importance of natural therapies in treating joint pain is highlighted in this section. It talks about the benefits they have over pharmaceutical choices, such as improved safety profiles. It also highlights how crucial an integrated strategy is for getting the best outcomes, combining conventional treatment and alternative medicines.

Readers will be inspired to investigate these options and discover more about their advantages in treating joint pain after realizing the significance of natural therapies and their capacity to provide significant alleviation.

People of all ages are often afflicted by joint discomfort, which may have a major negative influence on their quality of life. Joint pain may be uncomfortable, impair mobility, and interfere with everyday activities, regardless of the cause—it can be from an accident, age-related wear and tear, or a chronic illness like arthritis. Because of this, people who have joint pain often look for practical ways to reduce their discomfort and enhance their general health.

Growing evidence has been found in recent years supporting the value of natural treatments for joint pain. Natural pain reduction methods take a comprehensive approach to treating pain by enhancing general health and using the body's natural healing powers. These treatments come from plant-based ingredients including spices, herbs, and essential oils; they may also include modifying one's lifestyle to promote joint health.

Natural cures are significant not just because of their potential for success but also because they have less adverse effects than conventional pharmaceutical treatments. For people looking for safer and more gentle solutions, natural therapies are an enticing alternative to many traditional pain drugs, which might have negative side effects or long-term health concerns.

Furthermore, rather than only treating the symptoms, natural therapies for joint pain often target the underlying reasons of the condition. Beyond providing short-term comfort, they seek to strengthen the structure of the joints, lower inflammation, and enhance general joint health. This thorough introduction will delve into the realm of joint pain, examining its origins, symptoms, and the shortcomings of traditional treatment approaches. The importance of natural medicines will then be emphasized, along with their increasing potency and popularity. People might possibly improve their well-being and quality of life by managing their joint pain with educated judgments if they are aware of the benefits of natural therapies.

Chapter 1

Comprehending Arthritis

A prevalent condition that millions of individuals experience globally is joint discomfort. It may cause anything from mild discomfort to crippling agony, making daily tasks difficult. The goal of this thorough paper is to provide readers a full knowledge of joint pain, including typical forms, causes, risk factors, symptoms, and implications on day-to-day living.

Reasons and Danger Elements

Numerous things may lead to joint discomfort. The most frequent cause is arthritis, a disorder marked by joint inflammation. Among the major varieties of arthritis that may cause joint discomfort are gout, osteoarthritis, and rheumatoid arthritis.

Additional reasons might include joint damage or injuries including fractures, sprains, or strains. Joint pain may also result from infections, such as septic arthritis. In addition, a number of illnesses, including bursitis, fibromyalgia, and lupus, may aggravate joint discomfort.

There are many risk factors that raise the possibility of joint discomfort. Age is important since joint discomfort is more common in elderly persons. Due to the increased pressure that being overweight puts on the joints, obesity and a sedentary lifestyle both raise the risk of joint discomfort. Additionally, genetics may be involved, as some people may have a hereditary predisposition to joint discomfort.

Typical Types of Joint Pain

While every part in the body may experience joint pain, the knees, hips, shoulders, and hands are the most often afflicted. Every joint has a unique collection of structures and functions that might make it vulnerable to various kinds of pain.

The most common kind of arthritis, osteoarthritis, often affects joints that bear weight, such the knees and hips. Conversely, rheumatoid arthritis usually affects smaller joints, such as the hands and feet. The big toe joint is the main site of gout, which is characterized by abrupt, intense pain bouts.

Signs and Impact on Day-to-Day Activities

Depending on the underlying reason and severity of the problem, joint pain symptoms might change. Pain, edema, stiffness, redness, and a decreased range of motion in the afflicted joint are typical symptoms. In addition to causing weariness and weakening in the muscles, joint discomfort may also make it difficult to walk, lift items, or even put on clothes.

Joint discomfort may have a major effect on day-to-day activities. People who suffer from joint discomfort often find it difficult to move about and may need to use walkers or canes as assistance. As a result of the pain and diminished functionality, people with chronic joint pain may also experience an increase in stress, worry, and depression, which may worsen their mental health.

In summary, knowledge of joint pain is essential for people who are suffering it as well as those who provide care. Through an understanding of the origins, risk factors, common kinds, symptoms, and impact on day-to-day living, readers may have a greater understanding of the difficulties that people with joint pain encounter. To successfully manage joint pain and enhance overall quality of life, it is important to see a physician and investigate available treatment alternatives.

Chapter 2

Natural Treatments for Arthritis

All ages may be affected by the crippling illness known as joint pain. To maintain a good standard of living, it is essential to get effective treatment from any underlying ailments, whether they related to arthritis, injuries, or other disorders. Even though prescription drugs are often utilized, many people look for natural solutions to treat joint discomfort. We will discuss a variety of natural treatments in this extensive paper, such as herbal medicines, essential oils, nutritional supplements, and physical therapy that have had encouraging outcomes in reducing joint pain and enhancing mobility.

Herbal medicines: For millennia, people have used herbal medicines to treat a wide range of illnesses, including joint pain. These three well-liked herbal treatments have a reputation for being pain- and inflammation-relieving:

Turmeric: Curcumin, a substance found in turmeric, a bright yellow spice that is often used in Indian cooking, has potent anti-inflammatory properties. Curcumin is a useful natural treatment for joint pain since studies have shown how well it may relieve stiffness and soreness in the joints.

Ginger: Well-known for its digestive advantages, ginger also has anti-inflammatory qualities that may lessen joint discomfort. Gingerol, one of its active ingredients, is thought to lessen inflammation and increase joint flexibility. Reducing joint discomfort may be achieved by adding ginger to one's diet or by drinking ginger tea.

Indian frankincense, or boswellia, is a plant extract that has been used for generations in traditional medicine. Its anti-inflammatory qualities have been shown to successfully lessen joint discomfort and enhance joint functionality. Boswellia is often used topically or taken as a dietary supplement. It is available as capsules or cream.

Essential Oils: Plant-based essential oils are becoming more and more well-known for their many health advantages, which include their capacity to reduce joint pain. The following three essential oils have had encouraging outcomes:

Peppermint Oil: Peppermint oil includes menthol, a cooling substance that may help relieve inflammation and discomfort in the joints. By diluting a few drops in a carrier oil and rubbing it over the afflicted joints, it may be used topically.

Eucalyptus Oil: In addition to having an energizing aroma, eucalyptus oil has analgesic and anti-inflammatory qualities. Joint discomfort may be momentarily relieved by immediately applying eucalyptus oil to the afflicted regions.

Lavender Oil: Although its relaxing qualities are well-known, lavender oil also contains analgesic and anti-inflammatory qualities. Applying lavender oil to the joints may ease discomfort and encourage calmness.

Dietary Supplements: A number of dietary supplements have shown potential in easing joint discomfort and enhancing joint health. Consider the following three supplements:

Omega-3 Fatty Acids: Rich in flaxseed and fish oil, omega-3 fatty acids have anti-inflammatory qualities that may help lessen joint discomfort. The long-term advantages of omega-3 supplementation for joint health may be achieved by dietary changes.

Glucosamine and Chondroitin: These two naturally occurring substances are present in the cartilage of our joints. Their potential to lessen joint discomfort, increase mobility, and halt the development of osteoarthritis has been extensively researched.

Vitamin D: For the health of your bones and joints, vitamin D is essential. Sufficient amounts of vitamin D may aid in lowering joint discomfort and inflammation. For those with joint discomfort, making sure they get enough vitamin D from sunshine or supplements is crucial.

Physical treatments: Certain physical treatments have shown encouraging effects in the management of joint pain and enhancement of joint function, in addition to herbal medications and nutritional supplements. These are three well-liked choices:

Acupuncture: In order to reduce pain and enhance general health, ultra-thin needles are inserted into certain body locations. Acupuncture has been shown in several trials to be an effective means of reducing joint pain and improving mobility in patients with osteoarthritis and other joint diseases.

Hot and Cold Therapy: You may temporarily relieve joint pain and inflammation by applying heat or cold to the afflicted joints. While cold therapy—such as ice packs or cold compresses—reduces swelling and numbs the region, hot therapy—such as warm showers or heating pads—helps relax muscles and promote blood flow.

Massage treatment: Massage treatment is a useful tool for easing joint discomfort, lowering stress, and relaxing muscles. Massage treatment may enhance joint health by increasing flexibility, improving circulation, and promoting particular muscle groups with targeted pressure.

Natural joint pain management takes a comprehensive approach, addressing the root causes of suffering instead of just treating the symptoms. For those looking for nonpharmacological ways to relieve joint pain, herbal medicines, essential oils, nutritional supplements, and physical therapy are good substitutes for prescription drugs. Before implementing these treatments into your routine, you should, however, speak with a healthcare provider to be sure they are suitable for your particular ailment.

Chapter 3

Adjusting Your Lifestyle to Reduce Joint Pain and Achieve Your Best Health

Joint discomfort may be crippling and negatively affect your quality of life in general. Nonetheless, making some lifestyle adjustments may provide a great deal of comfort and support improved joint health. We will discuss four key lifestyle changes in this extensive paper that may help reduce joint discomfort, increase mobility, and improve your overall health.

Exercise and stretching: An active lifestyle that supports joint health must include regular exercise and stretching. Low-impact activities that increase flexibility and strengthen the muscles around your joints include walking, cycling, and swimming. Stretching techniques that increase joint mobility and decrease stiffness include yoga and Pilates. A physical therapist or other healthcare provider should be consulted in order to create a customized fitness program that takes into account your unique demands and restrictions.

Weight management: Reducing extra weight puts additional strain on your joints, especially the weight-bearing joints like your hips and knees. Therefore, maintaining a healthy weight is essential for relieving joint pain. You may lose weight gradually and sustainably by eating a healthy, balanced diet and getting frequent exercise. Speak with a qualified dietitian for advice on dietary changes that promote joint health, such as include foods high in antioxidants, omega-3 fatty acids, and other vitamins and minerals.

Dietary Adjustments: A few dietary adjustments might help lessen pain and inflammation in the joints. Natural pain treatment may be obtained by include anti-inflammatory foods in your regular meals, such as fatty fish (salmon, mackerel), nuts and seeds (walnuts, flaxseeds), fruits (berries, cherries), vegetables (spinach, kale), and spices (turmeric, ginger). Additionally, you may improve general joint health and minimize inflammation by cutting down on processed foods, refined sugars, and saturated fats in your diet.

Techniques for Stress Management: Prolonged stress may make joint discomfort worse and slow down the healing process. Consequently, using sensible stress-reduction strategies is essential for relieving joint discomfort. Take part in stress-relieving and relaxing activities, such mindfulness training, deep breathing techniques, or meditation. To reduce stress, one may also engage in regular physical exercise, spend time outside, and maintain a good work-life balance.

You may take proactive measures to control your joint pain and greatly enhance your general health by adopting these lifestyle modifications. Your muscles will become stronger and your joints will become more flexible with regular exercise and stretching, all while keeping your body healthy.

Chapter 4

Strategies for Preventing and Maintaining Optimal Health and Collaborative Assistance

In the fast-paced world of today, when bad posture and sedentary lifestyles are commonplace, it is critical to give preventative and maintenance methods top priority for our general health. This extensive essay examines several methods and approaches that may support general wellbeing, enhance posture, and preserve joint health. The most important things we can do to live a healthy and pain-free life are to include joint-friendly workouts, adopt good posture and body mechanics, make ergonomic changes, schedule routine check-ups, and maintain our health.

Exercises That Are Jointly Friendly

In maintaining joint health, physical activity is essential. But choosing the appropriate workouts is crucial to reducing wear and strain on joints and preventing accidents. Consider the following joint-friendly exercises:

1. **Low-impact aerobic workouts:** To keep your heart healthy without overstressing your joints, take up low-impact aerobic exercises like cycling, swimming, or walking.

2. **Strength training:** Increasing the strength of the muscles around your joints may improve stability and support. Exercises that target certain muscle groups should be prioritized, and good form and technique should be observed.

3. **Exercises for flexibility:** Include stretches to keep joints flexible and mobile. Pilates and yoga are great choices for improving alignment of the body and posture.

appropriate body mechanics and posture

Maintaining ideal musculoskeletal health and preventing chronic pain need good posture and body mechanics. Here are some pointers to help you with your body mechanics and posture:

1. **Sit and stand tall:** Keep your back straight, shoulders relaxed, and head balanced while sitting and standing to maintain a spine in alignment. Do not slump or bend forward.

2. **Ergonomic workstations:** Arrange the equipment in an ergonomic manner. To lessen joint strain, choose an adjustable chair with sufficient lumbar support, set your computer display at eye level, and keep your keyboard and mouse at a comfortable distance.

3. **Lift carefully:** Use your leg muscles and keep your spine in a neutral posture when you lift heavy things. When lifting, refrain from twisting or reaching too much.

Ergonomic Modifications

If our regular activities—such as sleeping, standing, and sitting—are not ergonomically adjusted, they might lead to joint tension. Take into account these ergonomic changes:

Ergonomic Changes: Improving Coziness and Productivity at Work

Taking care of our physical well-being is essential in the hectic and demanding work environment of today. Working for prolonged lengths of time may cause pain, exhaustion, and even long-term health problems. Ergonomic modifications are therefore relevant. We may lower our risk of musculoskeletal diseases (MSDs) and increase comfort and efficiency by making little changes to our workstations and behaviors. This post will discuss the value of ergonomic modifications and provide helpful advice for setting up an ergonomic workstation.

Comprehending Ergonomics: The study of how individuals interact with their workplace falls under the umbrella of ergonomics. It strives to maximize workstation layout and design to meet each person's demands while fostering productivity, comfort, and safety. Ergonomic modifications include rearranging our workstation, equipment, and personal habits and posture to minimize physical strain and enhance performance.

Advantages of Ergonomic Changes:

1. **Increased Comfort:** Ergonomic modifications reduce pain brought on by improper posture, repeated movements, or subpar gear. Our bodies may be appropriately aligned and supported as necessary to reduce strain on muscles, tendons, and joints, increasing comfort levels throughout the workday.

2. **Increased Efficiency:** We can work more effectively when our bodies are in the right positions. By streamlining the workflow and minimizing pointless motions, ergonomic modifications enable us to operate more accurately, productively, and with more attention.

3. **Prevention of Musculoskeletal Disorders** (MSDs): Neck strain, carpal tunnel syndrome, and back discomfort are examples of MSDs that may be brought on by poor ergonomics. Our long-term health may be protected and the likelihood of these problems reduced by making the appropriate ergonomic modifications.

Realistic Ergonomic Changes

1. **Sit Right:** Set your chair height so that your knees are 90 degrees from your feet and your feet are flat on the floor. If lumbar support is offered, place your back on the chair's backrest

as you sit. Remain calm in your posture; try not to slump or slant too far forward.

2. **Optimize workstation Setup:** Set up your workstation such that, while typing, your forearms are parallel to the floor. To reduce needless extending or reaching, keep commonly used things within arm's reach. To avoid straining your neck and eyes, keep reference materials in a document holder.

3. **Set Up Keyboard and Monitor:** Place your keyboard and monitor front and center.

Chapter 5

Revealing the Potential of Natural Treatments: Motivational Case Studies and Triumphs

In a society where synthetic drugs and fast fixes abound, natural treatments' effectiveness is sometimes underestimated. But as several success stories and real-world encounters have shown, nature has remarkable healing powers. We explore case studies and testimonies in this extensive essay, shedding light on the transformational potential of natural therapies. Come along on this fascinating trip as we examine the inspiring tales of people who have used natural therapies to achieve healing and rejuvenation.

Actual Experiences with Natural Solutions:

1. Using Herbal Therapies to Overcome Chronic Pain

Introducing Sarah, a dynamic lady who battled arthritis-related severe pain for years. Although the adverse effects of traditional therapies became a nuisance, they did provide temporary respite. Sarah became disillusioned with the cycle of drug use and looked for other solutions. By means of extensive investigation and individualized counseling with a herbalist, she found a customized concoction of herbs that progressively reduced her discomfort and swelling. Sarah is able to live an active life without being limited by her chronic pain because of the effectiveness of natural medicines.

2.   Using Probiotics to Restore Digestive Health

John was a fitness fanatic whose daily efforts were hampered by recurrent intestinal difficulties. He was given a variety of drugs and saw many physicians before discovering probiotics, which proved to be a game-changer in his life. When John started adding certain probiotic strains to his diet, his digestion and gut health significantly improved. His system's natural balance of healthy microorganisms not only reduced his symptoms but also improved his general health. John's experience serves as an excellent example of the enormous potential that natural therapies have for enhancing and repairing physiological processes.

3. Using Herbal Supplements and Mindfulness to Strengthen Mental Wellbeing]

Emma had constant tension and persistent worry. In search of a substitute for prescription drugs that caused her to feel disoriented and disoriented, she investigated the domain of mindfulness exercises and herbal remedies. Emma progressively saw a reduction in her anxiety symptoms by meditating regularly and adding adaptogenic herbs to her diet. In addition to providing a kind, compassionate approach to her mental health, the natural cures provided her a feeling of control over her own path to inner peace.

Examining Case Studies, Success Stories, and Actual Experiences with Natural Remedies to Unleash the Power of Nature.

We often find ourselves pulled to the marvels of nature in our pursuit of optimum health and wellbeing. Humanity has used natural treatments for ages to heal a wide range of illnesses and bring the body back into harmony. We're going to take a close look at case studies, success stories, and actual experiences with natural therapies today. In addition to providing information, our goal is to motivate you to pursue holistic well-being on your own.

Case Studies that Provided Clarity

Revisiting Nature's Prescription:

Nature has provided us with a plethora of powerful and efficient healing medicines. We reveal the therapeutic potential of plants, herbs, and other natural substances via engrossing case stories. These narratives explore the experiences of people who have found relief from conditions including chronic pain, sleep disturbances, anxiety, and digestive problems by turning to nature's pharmacy. To comprehend the workings and advantages of these natural medicines, we look at the scientific data supporting their experiences.

Analyzing the Intersection of contemporary Science and Ancient Wisdom: Natural treatments have endured because they connect contemporary scientific knowledge with ancient wisdom. We look at case studies that demonstrate the amazing convergence of evidence-based medicine with traditional healing methods. These tales demonstrate the great potential of natural treatments for ailments including mental clarity support, immune function enhancement, chronic condition management, and skin health promotion.

Success tales that Inspire Us to Move From Despair to Empowerment: We may be inspired and motivated by success tales. We tell the stories of people who have used natural treatments to go off on life-changing adventures. These stories demonstrate the triumph of the human spirit by presenting amazing recoveries from serious illnesses, lifestyle disorders, and psychological difficulties. We show the limitless possibilities that exist in the field of natural treatments by commemorating these successes.

Adopting a Holistic Lifestyle: Natural therapies provide a holistic lifestyle approach for flourishing well-being in addition to being effective in healing diseases. We share motivational stories of people who have realized the power of natural treatments to avoid illness, maintain young, and improve general vigor. These success stories demonstrate the transformational impact of a holistic approach, from taking herbal supplements to including mindful activities like yoga and meditation in their daily routines.

User Testimonials and Comments

The Strength of the People's Voice: Firsthand accounts attest to the efficacy and security of natural cures. We delve into illuminating testimonies and comments from those who have directly reaped the benefits of these treatments. Their first-hand experiences provide readers with direction and insightful information on the effectiveness, potential drawbacks, and general impacts of natural therapies on various medical issues.

Empowering Choices: We stress the significance of making well-informed decisions by showcasing a variety of testimonies. Readers are able to make well-informed decisions suited to their own requirements by gaining a thorough grasp of how others have employed natural therapies to address certain difficulties. These firsthand accounts show how natural therapies may support traditional medical care while enabling people to take control of their health.

The exploration's case studies, success stories, and firsthand accounts highlight the enormous potential of natural medicines. The life-changing experiences of those who have experienced nature's healing power inspire us as readers. Equipped with information and bolstered by firsthand experiences, we set out on our own journey toward comprehensive wellness, combining forces with the wisdom of nature to live a more vibrant, healthier life.

Chapter 6

Enhance Your Knowledge: Exploring Additional Resources and References

In today's ever-evolving world, the pursuit of knowledge is an ongoing journey. While we often rely on traditional sources such as books and journals, the advent of the internet has opened up a plethora of additional resources and references. In this comprehensive note, we will explore various avenues to expand our understanding, including books, journals, research papers, websites, online communities, as well as professional organizations and associations. By leveraging these resources, you can bolster your knowledge and connect with like-minded individuals who share your passions and interests.

Books, Journals, and Research Papers:

Books have long been treasured sources of information and inspiration. They provide in-depth analyses, expert perspectives, and valuable insights into specific topics. Whether you prefer physical copies or digital formats, books offer an immersive way to delve into subjects of interest.

When it comes to scholarly work, journals and research papers are invaluable resources. Academic journals contain peer-reviewed articles that contribute to the knowledge base within a particular field. Research papers, on the other hand, present groundbreaking research findings and enable you to stay updated with the latest advancements. Libraries, online databases, and academic platforms are great places to access these resources, including platforms like JSTOR, PubMed, and Google Scholar.

Websites and Online Communities:

The internet has revolutionized the availability of information, offering endless opportunities to access a wide range of resources conveniently. Websites dedicated to various topics provide a wealth of knowledge, research, and practical insights. When exploring online content, it's crucial to use reputable sources and critically evaluate the information.

Online communities and forums centered around specific interests allow individuals to connect, discuss, and share ideas. Platforms like Reddit, Quora, and Stack Exchange provide communities that foster engagement with experts and enthusiasts alike. Engaging in these communities can expand your understanding through discussions, learning from others, and seeking guidance on complex subjects.

Furthermore, websites like TED Talks, Khan Academy, and Coursera offer video lectures, tutorials, and courses from industry professionals and leading experts. These platforms provide an interactive and engaging way to learn new skills and gain a deeper understanding of diverse topics.

Professional Organizations and Associations:

Joining professional organizations and associations related to your field of interest can be an incredible asset to your knowledge-building journey. These groups provide access to conferences, seminars, workshops, and publications specifically tailored to advance knowledge and drive professional growth.

Professional organizations and associations play a crucial role in enhancing and supporting various industries and sectors. These organizations bring together like-minded professionals, fostering a sense of community, knowledge sharing, networking, and continuous professional development. By joining such organizations, individuals gain access to a wide range of resources, opportunities, and connections that can significantly enhance their careers. Here, we explore the importance and benefits of professional organizations and associations.

1. **Networking Opportunities:**

One of the greatest benefits of joining professional organizations and associations is the networking opportunities they provide. These organizations bring together professionals from the same field or industry, creating a platform for collaboration, idea exchange, and relationship building. Networking within these communities can lead to new business partnerships, mentorship opportunities, job prospects, and the sharing of best practices.

2. **Continued Professional Development:**

Professional organizations and associations are committed to promoting and advancing their respective fields. They offer numerous opportunities for members to develop their skills, knowledge, and expertise through workshops, seminars, conferences, webinars, and other learning events. These resources ensure that members stay updated with the latest industry trends, advancements, and regulatory changes, which is crucial for professional growth and staying competitive in today's fast-paced world.

3. **Access to Resources and Information:**

Belonging to a professional organization provides access to an extensive range of resources and information that might not be readily available elsewhere. These organizations often offer repositories of research papers, industry reports, case studies, and other valuable publications. They may also provide members with exclusive access to online forums, discussion boards, and member directories, facilitating information sharing, problem-solving, and collaboration.

4. Advocacy and Policy Influence:

Professional organizations and associations often play an essential role in advocating for their industries and professionals on important issues. They voice collective concerns, promote policy changes, and represent their members' interests at the local, national, and international levels. Through their influence and lobbying efforts, these organizations can have a significant impact on shaping regulations, standards, and practices that affect their respective fields.

5. Career Advancement:

Being an active member in a professional organization can enhance one's career prospects significantly. Membership in these organizations demonstrates a commitment to professional excellence and ongoing development, which can be an attractive quality for employers. Additionally, many associations offer career services such as job boards, resume reviews, and interview preparation resources, providing members with valuable support during job searches and career transitions.

6. **Peer Recognition and Professional Credibility:**

Being associated with a reputable professional organization adds credibility to an

Chapter 7

CONCLUSION

A prevalent ailment that impacts millions of individuals globally is joint discomfort. It may have a major negative effect on someone's quality of life by impairing their movement and making them uncomfortable. This article has discussed a number of natural treatments, lifestyle modifications, and preventative techniques that may help reduce joint discomfort and improve joint health in general.

We covered a thorough overview of natural treatments for joint pain in the first segment. Natural solutions provide a comprehensive method of treating joint pain without the possible negative effects of prescription drugs. We spoke about the advantages of include foods high in anti-inflammatory compounds in one's diet, such green tea, ginger, turmeric, and omega-3 fatty acids, which are present in flaxseed and fish. In order to lessen the load on the joints, we also emphasized the need of maintaining a healthy weight via exercise and a balanced diet. We also looked into the possible help offered by alternative treatments such as massage, acupuncture, and herbal supplements.

The second part summarized preventive techniques and lifestyle modifications that may support joint health. We underlined the importance of consistent exercise in enhancing flexibility and range of motion as well as strengthening the muscles around the joints. For those who have joint discomfort, low-impact exercises like yoga, cycling, and swimming might be very helpful. We also emphasized how crucial it is to use ergonomic equipment and keep proper posture in order to reduce joint tension. In addition, as stress may exacerbate the symptoms of joint pain, we also spoke about the effects of stress-reduction practices on joint health, such as mindfulness and meditation.

In conclusion, we encouraged you to consult a specialist. Many people find that natural treatments and lifestyle modifications help them manage their joint pain, but for a thorough assessment and individualized treatment plan, it is essential to speak with a healthcare provider, such as an orthopedic specialist or rheumatologist. These experts are able to provide precise diagnoses, suggest suitable drugs when needed, and give customized therapy based on the requirements of the client.

In conclusion, joint pain is a common problem that may be resolved and joint health improved by using natural therapies, making lifestyle adjustments, and seeing a specialist. It's important to keep in mind that every person's path to treating joint pain is different, and it might take some trial and error to discover the ideal mix of treatments and tactics. A life with less joint pain and more mobility is achievable with perseverance and a thorough strategy.